THE GODDESS METHOD:

Unlocking Optimal Health and Blood Sugar Balance, Cutting Cravings, Getting Your Energy Back, and Feeling Amazing, with a 4-Week Guide

Contents

INTRODUCTION 3

CHAPTER 1: UNDERSTANDING
BLOOD SUGAR IMBALANCES.................5

THE IMPORTANCE OF BLOOD
SUGAR REGULATION 5

COMMON CAUSES OF BLOOD
SUGAR IMBALANCES 8

THE IMPACT OF BLOOD SUGAR ON
OVERALL HEALTH 10

CHAPTER 2: THE SCIENCE BEHIND
GLUCOSE REGULATION 13

HOW GLUCOSE METABOLISM
WORKS..13

HORMONES ARE INVOLVED IN
BLOOD SUGAR REGULATION.........16

THE ROLE OF INSULIN AND
GLUCAGON..19

How insulin works 20

How glucagon works.........................21

CHAPTER 3: ASSESSING YOUR BLOOD
SUGAR HEALTH....................................23

BLOOD SUGAR TESTING AND MONITORING 23

Why test your blood sugar? 23

When to test your blood sugar 24

Type 1 diabetes 24

Type 2 diabetes 25

What if you have a continuous glucose monitor (CGM)? 26

Know your target range. 28

How to test your blood sugar 29

INTERPRETING BLOOD SUGAR RESULTS 31

IDENTIFYING PATTERNS AND TRIGGERS 33

CHAPTER 4: 35

THE GLUCOSE GODDESS NUTRITION PLAN 35

BALANCING MACRONUTRIENTS FOR STABLE BLOOD SUGAR 35

FOODS TO INCLUDE AND AVOID . 39

MEAL PLANNING AND PORTION CONTROL..................................40

CHAPTER 5: 44

EXERCISE AND PHYSICAL ACTIVITY44

THE IMPACT OF EXERCISE ON BLOOD SUGAR...................................44

EXERCISE SIGNIFICANTLY IMPACTS BLOOD SUGAR...................................47

CREATING AN EXERCISE ROUTINE 49

CHAPTER 6: 54

STRESS MANAGEMENT AND BLOOD SUGAR 54

UNDERSTANDING THE STRESS-BLOOD SUGAR CONNECTION.........54

STRESS REDUCTION TECHNIQUES 58

INCORPORATING MINDFULNESS AND RELAXATION PRACTICES 61

CHAPTER 7: 65

LIFESTYLE MODIFICATIONS FOR BALANCED BLOOD SUGAR 65

SLEEP AND BLOOD SUGAR REGULATION 65

HYDRATION AND BLOOD SUGAR HEALTH 66

STRATEGIES FOR LONG-TERM SUCCESS 70

CHAPTER 8: TROUBLESHOOTING AND DEALING WITH CHALLENGES . 73

HANDLING BLOOD SUGAR FLUCTUATIONS 73

It Can Be Prevented Through: 74

COPING WITH CRAVINGS AND TEMPTATIONS 76

CONCLUSION 80

DISCLAIMER

This book is as accurate and complete as possible. There may be typographical errors or mistakes in the content. This book also contains information that is only current as of the publication date. This Book is not the definitive source of information and should only be used as a guide. The book's sole purpose is to teach. The publisher or author does not guarantee the eBook's accuracy. They are not responsible for any error, omissions, or misinformation.

INTRODUCTION

We hope you enjoy your time at "The Glucose Goddess Method"! This ground-breaking book will equip you with the knowledge and skills necessary to take control of your health and achieve a state of balanced blood sugar levels. This technique, based on an in-depth comprehension of the significance of glucose control, provides a comprehensive approach to managing your blood sugar levels and transforming your general well-being.

Keeping stable blood sugar levels in today's fast-paced environment can be a big problem for those who struggle with diabetes. Blood sugar imbalances may have far-reaching implications for several parts of our lives, including our energy levels, ability to control our weight, mood, and general vitality, and the Glucose Goddess Method recognizes this fact. This program enables you to take charge of your health and live your life to the fullest by addressing the underlying causes of these imbalances and giving practical techniques. Its goal is to empower you to live your life to the fullest.

The Glucose Goddess Method equips you with the resources, information, and support you need to accomplish the long-lasting outcomes you desire, regardless of whether you are battling prediabetes or diabetes or want to maximize your well-being. Put an end to the wild ride of unpredictable blood sugar levels and take the first step toward a more vibrant and balanced life.

With the help of The Glucose Goddess Method, you are about to embark on a life-changing adventure that will lead you to become the most amazing version of yourself. Get ready to make this happen! Let's find out how to harness the power of stable blood sugar levels and enjoy a life full of vitality, energy, and overall well-being as a group.

CHAPTER 1: UNDERSTANDING BLOOD SUGAR IMBALANCES

THE IMPORTANCE OF BLOOD SUGAR REGULATION

One's general health and well-being must keep their blood sugar levels steady. The sugar in our blood, also called glucose, serves as the principal fuel for the cells and tissues in our body. When our blood sugar levels are stable, we have better control over our moods, increased cognitive function, and consistent energy.

However, disrupting the normal amounts of sugar in the blood can cause various health problems. The presence of illnesses such as diabetes, characterized by persistently high blood sugar levels, can cause long-term damage to blood vessels and organs, elevating the risk of heart disease, stroke, and other consequences. Conversely, low blood sugar levels, often known as hypoglycemia, can bring on symptoms such as dizziness, weakness, and in extreme cases, even loss of consciousness.

People's ability to establish optimal blood sugar balance and to keep it over time is the goal of the Glucose Goddess Method, which was devised to assist them. This comprehensive strategy considers all areas of health, such as eating well, being physically active, maintaining healthy lifestyle choices, and learning to cope with stress. By making some straightforward adjustments to these aspects of your life, you may facilitate an atmosphere favorable to maintaining healthy blood sugar levels, which are essential for maintaining your overall health.

Managing blood sugar is absolutely necessary to effectively operate all major bodily systems. The health of one's brain, adrenal glands, immunological system, thyroid, and digestive system are all significantly impacted by blood sugar levels. Chronic dysglycemia, an inability to properly regulate blood sugar, has been linked to an increased risk of obesity, hormonal imbalances, adrenal fatigue, hypothyroidism, and other conditions. Concerning dysglycemia, the two most important issues to look out for are hypoglycemia and insulin resistance.

Hypoglycemia refers to abnormally low blood sugar levels. In most cases, this occurs as a response to an increase in insulin levels brought on by consuming a meal heavy in sugar or carbohydrates. These insulin surges and accompanying glucose reductions are troublesome if they occur regularly throughout the day, causing blood sugar levels to fluctuate from high to low. The difficulty arises when these insulin surges and following glucose drops repeatedly occur throughout the day. Suppose you miss meals or do not consume sufficient amounts of protein and fat as fuel, instead relying solely on sugary foods. In that case, you will experience frequent dips in your energy level and cognitive performance.

On the other side, if you consistently consume an unhealthy quantity of sugar, your body will have to produce excessive insulin to digest the glucose and deliver it to the cells in your body. After sufficient time, the body will eventually reach a point where it will no longer take this message seriously and begin to disregard the signal. As a result, the cells will grow resistant to insulin. When glucose, which is needed to supply energy to the cells, cannot enter the cells, basic cellular functioning breaks down, symptoms appear, and the body stores the extra sugar as fat.

COMMON CAUSES OF BLOOD SUGAR IMBALANCES

Understanding the factors contributing to blood sugar imbalances is crucial for effective management. Several lifestyle and dietary factors can disrupt blood sugar regulation, such as:

- Unhealthy Diet: Consuming sugary and processed foods can lead to sudden spikes in blood sugar levels and subsequent crashes, stressing the body's insulin response.

- Sedentary Lifestyle: Lack of physical activity can lead to insulin resistance, making it harder for cells to utilize glucose effectively.
- Chronic Stress: When stressed, the body releases hormones like cortisol, which can raise blood sugar levels.
- Poor Sleep: Inadequate sleep can negatively impact insulin sensitivity and disrupt glucose metabolism.
- Genetics: Family history and genetic factors can affect an individual's susceptibility to blood sugar imbalances.

The Glucose Goddess Method offers a comprehensive approach to managing blood sugar imbalances, including nutrition, lifestyle, and mindset interventions. By making small changes to diet and lifestyle habits, it's possible to support the body's natural ability to regulate blood sugar levels and reduce the intensity of imbalances. Additionally, The Glucose

Goddess Method emphasizes cultivating self-compassion and embracing your unique needs to make sustainable progress towards wellness. With this holistic approach, you can begin living with ease around food again.

If you're curious about how The Glucose Goddess Method might be able to help you find balance in your life, don't hesitate to reach out for more information! You deserve to experience vitality and stability without sacrificing your health. Reach out today, and let's get started on your journey toward optimum health. Together, we'll make it happen!

THE IMPACT OF BLOOD SUGAR ON OVERALL HEALTH

The effects of blood sugar imbalances extend beyond diabetes and its immediate symptoms. Chronically high blood sugar levels can lead to a condition known as metabolic syndrome, characterized by a cluster of risk factors that increase the likelihood of heart disease, stroke, and type 2 diabetes.

Blood sugar fluctuations can also impact cognitive function, affecting concentration, memory, and mood stability. Many individuals may experience irritability, mood swings, and fatigue due to unstable blood sugar levels.

Moreover, blood sugar imbalances can disrupt the body's ability to manage weight effectively. Elevated blood sugar levels can lead to increased fat storage and hinder weight loss efforts, making it challenging for some individuals to achieve their health and fitness goals.
By recognizing the significance of blood sugar regulation, individuals can take proactive steps to improve their overall health and prevent potential complications. The Glucose Goddess Method is designed to address these concerns holistically, offering practical strategies and personalized guidance to help you achieve balanced blood sugar levels and enhance your quality of life.

By integrating mindful lifestyle changes and a customized nutrition plan, the Glucose Goddess Method provides a comprehensive approach to health that can improve blood sugar levels and support long-term well-being. Start your journey today with personalized guidance from The Glucose Goddess!

The Glucose Goddess Method prioritizes lasting change over quick fixes, so you can get on the path to improved health without sacrificing delicious food or an active lifestyle. Through interactive tools and regular check-ins with a certified nutrition coach, it helps you stay on track while uncovering the root causes of blood sugar dysregulation to address them effectively.

CHAPTER 2: THE SCIENCE BEHIND GLUCOSE REGULATION

HOW GLUCOSE METABOLISM WORKS

Understanding the process of glucose metabolism is key to understanding blood sugar regulation. When we consume carbohydrates, our digestive system breaks them down into glucose, which enters the bloodstream. Glucose is then transported to various cells throughout the body to provide energy for their functioning.

A delicate balance between glucose uptake and utilization is necessary to maintain stable blood sugar levels. The pancreas' hormone insulin plays a crucial role in this procedure. Insulin acts as a "key" that unlocks cells, allowing glucose to enter and be used for energy production.

Once inside the cells, glucose undergoes a series of metabolic reactions, producing ATP (adenosine triphosphate), the body's primary energy currency. Insulin also helps store excess glucose in the liver and muscles as glycogen for later use.

In contrast, the hormone glucagon, also produced by the pancreas, helps raise blood sugar levels when they are too low. Glucagon triggers the breakdown of stored glycogen into glucose, which is then released into the bloodstream, ensuring a constant energy supply.

Glucagon works to counterbalance the actions of insulin.
About 4–6 hours after you eat, the glucose levels in your blood decrease.
This triggers your pancreas to produce glucagon.
This hormone signals your liver and muscle cells to convert the stored glycogen into glucose. These cells then release the glucose into your bloodstream, so your other cells can use it for energy.
This whole feedback loop with insulin and glucagon is constantly in motion. It keeps your blood sugar levels from dipping too low, ensuring your body has a steady energy supply.

The Glucose Goddess Method takes this balancing act a step further. It teaches you how to use the power of food, lifestyle, and mindset changes to help maintain stable blood sugar levels. By eating the right types of carbohydrates at the right times and incorporating mindful movement into your day, you can unlock your body's natural ability to regulate insulin production and optimize glucose metabolism. The result? More life energy – without leaving you feeling drained or foggy-headed after meals. With an understanding of how the body uses glucose, we can work together to help create balance in your system! This will not only boost energy levels but also support overall health. So dive in and enjoy the journey with us! Let's get started on the Glucose Goddess Method!

The Glucose Goddess Method will help you:
• Gain an understanding of how carbs, proteins, and fats interact with your body to create balance
• Identify which foods work best for your unique needs

• Incorporate mindful movement into your daily routine
• Balance hormones and manage stress levels
• Make lifestyle changes that support blood sugar stability

With this knowledge, you can make informed food choices and develop a deeper appreciation for how food affects our bodies. With guidance from the Glucose Goddess Method, you will be empowered to take control of your health and live life to its fullest!

HORMONES ARE INVOLVED IN BLOOD SUGAR REGULATION

In addition to insulin and glucagon, several other hormones play crucial roles in blood sugar regulation:

- Cortisol: The adrenal glands' release of this stress hormone causes the liver to release glucose from its reserves, which can raise blood sugar levels.

- Epinephrine and Norepinephrine: These hormones, commonly known as adrenaline and noradrenaline, are released during stress or in response to a threat. They raise blood sugar levels by stimulating glycogen breakdown and inhibiting insulin release.
- Growth hormone, which the pituitary gland produces, promotes lipolysis (the breakdown of fats) and gluconeogenesis (the production of glucose from non-carbohydrate sources), helping maintain blood sugar levels during fasting.
- Incretins: These hormones, such as GLP-1 (glucagon-like peptide 1) and GIP (glucose-dependent insulinotropic peptide), are released from the intestines after meals. They increase insulin secretion, which helps cells take up glucose.
- Leptin: Known as the "satiety hormone," leptin helps regulate appetite and body weight. It also influences insulin sensitivity and glucose metabolism.

Thyroid hormones: The thyroid gland's T3 and T4 hormones help maintain blood sugar levels by increasing insulin sensitivity. They also promote glycogen synthesis, which helps store glucose for energy.

By understanding the roles of these hormones in regulating blood sugar, practitioners can use the Glucose Goddess Method to support their clients' health goals. This approach to managing blood sugar includes lifestyle modifications such as healthy eating, regular physical activity, and stress reduction. Additionally, dietary supplements like chromium, magnesium, and vanadium can support healthy blood sugar levels alongside a tailored exercise program. These interventions work together to balance out the body's hormones that affect blood sugar regulation—keeping individuals feeling their best!

Ultimately, the Glucose Goddess Method is a comprehensive approach to understanding and managing blood sugar levels. With proper lifestyle modifications, dietary supplements, and exercise programs tailored to each individual's needs, clients can be empowered with the tools they need to support their health goals and maintain optimal blood sugar balance.

THE ROLE OF INSULIN AND GLUCAGON

Insulin and glucagon work in a delicate balance to maintain blood sugar homeostasis. When blood sugar levels rise after a meal, the pancreas releases insulin, signaling cells to take up glucose and store it as glycogen or use it for energy. Insulin also inhibits glucagon release, preventing the liver from releasing stored glucose. Conversely, when blood sugar levels drop, the pancreas reduces insulin production, releasing glucagon. Glucagon triggers the breakdown of stored glycogen into glucose, released into the bloodstream to raise blood sugar levels.

This intricate dance between insulin and glucagon ensures blood sugar levels stay within a narrow range, providing a steady energy supply to the body's cells. Understanding the intricate science behind glucose regulation helps us appreciate the complexity of maintaining balanced blood sugar levels. By gaining insights into the hormonal interplay and metabolic processes involved, we can make informed choices and adopt strategies to support optimal blood sugar management. The Glucose Goddess Method harnesses this knowledge to empower individuals with effective tools and techniques for achieving and sustaining balanced blood sugar levels.

How insulin works

The body's cells need glucose for energy; insulin enables glucose to enter the cells. Insulin attaches Trusted Source
 To insulin receptors on cells throughout the body, instructing them to open and grant entry to glucose.

Low levels of insulin constantly circulate throughout the body. A spike in insulin signals the liver that a person's blood glucose level is also high, causing the liver to absorb glucose and change it into glycogen.

When blood sugar levels drop, glucagon instructs the liver to convert the glycogen back to glucose, causing a person's blood sugar levels to return to normal.

How glucagon works

The liver stores glucose to power cells during periods of low blood sugar. Skipping meals and getting inadequate nutrition can lower blood sugar levels. By storing glucose, the liver ensures the body's blood glucose levels remain steady between meals and during sleep.

When a person's blood glucose levels fall, pancreatic cells secrete glucagon, stimulating gluconeogenesis and glycogenolysis. The liver provides a trusted Source

Or stimulates the production of glucose using these processes.

In glycogenolysis, glucagon instructs the liver to convert glycogen to glucose, making glucose more available in the bloodstream.

In gluconeogenesis, the liver produces glucose from the byproducts of other processes. Gluconeogenesis also occurs in the kidneys and some other organs.

When the body's glucose levels rise, insulin moves the glucose into cells.

Insulin and glucagon work in a cycle. Glucagon interacts with the liver to increase blood sugar, while insulin reduces blood sugar by helping the cells use glucose.

CHAPTER 3: ASSESSING YOUR BLOOD SUGAR HEALTH

BLOOD SUGAR TESTING AND MONITORING

If you have diabetes, self-testing your blood sugar (blood glucose) can be important in managing diabetes and preventing complications. You can use a device called a continuous glucose monitor (CGM). Or you can test your blood sugar at home with a portable electronic device called a blood sugar meter using a small drop of your blood.

Why test your blood sugar?

Blood sugar testing provides useful information for diabetes management. It can help you:

- Monitor the effect of diabetes medications on blood sugar levels
- Identify blood sugar levels that are high or low

- Track your progress in reaching your overall treatment goals
- Learn how diet and exercise affect blood sugar levels
- Understand how other factors, such as illness or stress, affect blood sugar levels

When to test your blood sugar

Your healthcare provider will tell you how often to check your blood sugar levels. The testing frequency usually depends on the type of diabetes you have and your treatment plan.

Type 1 diabetes

Your health care provider may recommend blood sugar testing 4 to 10 times daily if you have type 1 diabetes. You may need to test:

- Before meals and snacks
- Before and after exercise
- Before bed

- During the night (sometimes),
- More often, if you're ill
- More often, if you change your daily routine
- More often, if you start a new medication,

Type 2 diabetes

If you take insulin to manage type 2 diabetes, your healthcare provider may recommend blood sugar testing several times a day, depending on the type and amount of insulin you use. If you take multiple daily injections, testing is usually recommended before meals and bedtime. You may need to test only before breakfast and sometimes before dinner or at bedtime if you use just an intermediate- or long-acting insulin.

If you manage type 2 diabetes with noninsulin medications or with diet and exercise alone, you may not need to test your blood sugar daily.

What if you have a continuous glucose monitor (CGM)?

CGMs are an option for those with diabetes, particularly type 1 diabetes, who want to monitor their blood sugar levels. These gadgets use a sensor implanted under the skin to read the user's blood sugar every few minutes. Before needing to be replaced, these sensors are normally worn for one to two weeks.

The most recent innovation in continuous glucose monitoring is a sensor that can be implanted under the skin and monitor blood sugar levels for three months. Blood sugar information is wirelessly transmitted from a sensor to an app on a smartphone through a transmitter worn on the body.

Some systems constantly display your current blood sugar reading on a receiver, smartphone, or wristwatch, and they sound an alert if your blood sugar level is rising or falling too rapidly for the gadget to handle. Some models require you to self-monitor your blood sugar levels regularly, bypassing the receiver over the sensor.

To calibrate the equipment, most of these devices still require finger-stick examinations. Check the user's handbook for your device to see whether or not you are required to check and, if so, how frequently you are required to do so.

Albuterol (ProAir HFA, Ventolin HFA, and others), acetaminophen (Tylenol, and others), and lisinopril (Prinivil, Zestril, and others) are just a few examples of drugs that have the potential to affect the accuracy of some CGM readings. This is especially true for earlier types of CGMs. Standard dosages of acetaminophen, up to 1,000 milligrams for an adult, do not appear to affect the readings produced by more recent CGMs.

If you are required to take drugs that might alter the readings' accuracy, your doctor may advise you to verify the results of your CGM with a regular blood sugar meter. Suppose you are pregnant, receiving dialysis, or in a severe condition. In that case, you should discuss wearing a CGM with your primary care physician before doing so, as these factors may impact the blood sugar readings that a CGM provides.

Know your target range.

Ask your healthcare provider for a reasonable blood sugar range. Your healthcare provider will set target blood sugar test results based on several factors, including:

- Type and severity of diabetes
- Age
- How long you lived with diabetes?
- Pregnancy status
- The presence of diabetes complications
- Overall health and the presence of other medical conditions

The American Diabetes Association (ADA) generally recommends the following target blood sugar levels:

- Between 80 and 130 milligrams per deciliter (mg/dL) or 4.4 and 7.2 millimoles per liter (mmol/L) before meals
- Less than 180 mg/dL (10.0 mmol/L) two hours after meals

But the ADA notes that these goals often vary depending on your age and personal health and should be individualized. Some people will have slightly higher blood sugar goals, including people who:

- Are age 60 and older
- Have other medical conditions, such as heart, lung, or kidney disease
- Have a reduced ability to sense low blood sugar levels (hypoglycemia unawareness)

How to test your blood sugar

Blood sugar testing requires the use of a blood sugar meter. The meter measures the amount of sugar in a small blood sample, usually from your fingertip, that you place on a disposable test strip. Even if you use a CGM, you'll still need a blood sugar meter to calibrate your device daily.

Your healthcare provider or certified diabetes care and education specialist can recommend an appropriate device. He or she can also help you learn how to use your meter.
Follow the instructions that come with your blood sugar meter. In general, here's how the process works:

1. Wash and dry your hands well. (Food and other substances can give you an inaccurate reading.)
2. Insert a test strip into your meter.
3. Prick the side of your fingertip with the needle (lancet) provided with your test kit.
4. Touch and hold the edge of the test strip against the drop of blood.
5. After a few seconds, the meter will display your blood sugar level on a screen.

Some meters can test blood taken from an alternate site, such as the forearm or palm.

But these readings may not be as accurate as readings from the fingertips, especially after a meal or during exercise, when blood sugar levels change more frequently. Alternate sites aren't recommended for use in calibrating CGMs.

INTERPRETING BLOOD SUGAR RESULTS

The Glucose Goddess Method of Interpreting Blood Sugar Results combines quantitative analysis and qualitative, subjective evaluation. Blood glucose readings are reflected on the scale as percentages, which provide an objective numerical representation for health professionals to use in diagnosing diabetes and monitoring its progression over time. The Glucose Goddess Method goes beyond that by taking into account the patient's experience with their symptoms, such as fatigue or hunger, to create a more comprehensive understanding of what is happening within their body. This method also looks at pre- and post-meal numbers to help identify potential causes of fluctuations in blood sugars. By combining objective and subjective data into one informal report, healthcare providers can get a clearer picture of how well-controlled someone's diabetes is and whether any underlying issues need to be addressed. The individual can also use this approach to understand their health better and identify possible improvement areas for overall wellness. The Glucose Goddess Method helps people take an active role in managing their diabetes rather than relying solely on healthcare professionals.

By taking a holistic approach to interpreting blood sugar results, this method provides a more accurate assessment of how well-controlled someone's diabetes is, ultimately leading to improved outcomes for those living with the condition. Additionally, it can help individuals develop healthier lifestyle habits that will benefit them over time and reduce long-term complications caused by uncontrolled diabetes. So if you're looking for a comprehensive way to monitor your diabetes, consider the Glucose Goddess Method. It could be just what you need to understand and manage your condition to stay healthy!

Although the Glucose Goddess Method is not a replacement for traditional glucose testing or healthcare visits, it can be an invaluable tool in helping individuals take charge of their diabetes management. With its combination of objective and subjective data, this method allows individuals to comprehensively understand their health, identify issues early on, and make any necessary lifestyle changes accordingly. So if you're looking for a new way to monitor your diabetes, try the Glucose Goddess Method today! You won't regret it.

IDENTIFYING PATTERNS AND TRIGGERS

The Glucose Goddess Method goes beyond just tracking food intake and glucose levels. It also encourages individuals to pay attention to patterns in their blood sugar levels and any potential triggers causing them to fluctuate. By identifying these patterns and triggers, individuals can make more informed decisions about foods they should (and should not) eat to stabilize their blood sugar.

Additionally, the Glucose Goddess Method encourages individuals to experiment with different types of meals and snacks, allowing them to find out what works best for their unique bodies. This can help people manage their diabetes over time by ensuring a balanced diet that checks their blood sugars.

Ultimately, the Glucose Goddess Method is an empowering approach to diabetes management that can help individuals take control of their health and create a plan that works for them. With the right tools and knowledge, anyone can live a healthier life with diabetes!

CHAPTER 4:

THE GLUCOSE GODDESS NUTRITION PLAN

BALANCING MACRONUTRIENTS FOR STABLE BLOOD SUGAR

There are six essential nutrients we need for survival, and they are broken down into two categories:

A. carbohydrates, fats, and protein.
B. Micronutrients: Water, minerals, and vitamins.
We need A to utilize and absorb B properly, all of us to thrive in life! Stay with me here. After breaking them into two categories, let's break them down individually by their functions.

A. Carbohydrates: These are the main source of energy for our brain. Without them, our bodies can not function properly or well.

Examples include Fruits, veggies, whole grains, and sugars.

B. Fats: Fat is the body's most condensed energy source. Consumption increases the absorption of micronutrients, including vitamins A, D, K, and E. Proper fat consumption is important to manufacture biochemicals such as hormones.
Examples include Nuts, seeds, rich omega-3 fish like salmon, healthy oils, and avocado.

C. Protein is the major structural component of cells and is responsible for repairing body tissues. Protein is broken down into amino acids, which are the building blocks of protein. Nine are not synthesized in our bodies, so they are essential to get from eating protein.
Examples include free-range meat, dairy, beans, eggs, and seeds.

D. Water makes up 75% of our bodies. It's extremely important to maintain homeostasis and transport nutrients to cells. It assists in removing waste products from the body. The best way to get it is to drink it, though many foods are high in water. We recommend drinking around 80 oz a day or MORE!

E. Minerals: Minerals help regulate cellular function. They help your body grow, develop, and stay healthy. Oftentimes, deficiency can lead to disease. These can be obtained mostly from food and sometimes need to be supplemented.

F. Vitamins: These are very important to overall health, development, and growth on every level in the body. Vitamin C supports the synthesis of collagen. Vitamin D helps maintain homeostasis, sustain energy, and improve cellular function. These can typically be attained on a 2000-calorie diet. Sometimes, you need to supplement.

The purpose of explaining the SIX essential nutrients was to explain further the proper way of combining them to achieve optimal health and weight and fight most diseases. Our entire teaching has been based on the stable blood sugar philosophy. When properly pairing your carbohydrates with fat and protein, you will continue to burn fat for fuel all day. By eating the correct ratios of carbohydrates, fat, and protein, you experience healthy energy and brain functioning. You avoid vitamin and mineral deficiencies when you eat the proper amount of these macronutrients. Make sense?

The general ratio we teach our clients to eat is:
50% carbohydrates
20% protein
30% fat

This general rule can vary by a few percentages depending on certain goals the individual is trying to attain.

The way to achieve healthy blood sugar is to follow these guidelines:
1. Eat within an hour of waking up
2. Eat every 2-4 hours during the day
3. ALWAYS combine all THREE macronutrients

FOODS TO INCLUDE AND AVOID

1 . Foods to Include:

- Complex carbohydrates such as oats, quinoa, sweet potatoes, and legumes
- Lean proteins such as chicken, turkey, fish, and egg whites
- Healthy fats, including avocado, olive oil, nuts and seeds, and nut and seed butter
- Low glycemic fruits like berries and apples
- Non-starchy vegetables such as spinach, kale, bell peppers, and cauliflower

2. Foods to Avoid:

- Refined grains such as white bread and pasta
- Sugary snacks like candy bars or cookies
- High-fat meats such as bacon or sausage
- Processed foods that contain artificial sweeteners or preservatives
- Dried fruits high in sugar, such as raisins and dates
- Deep-fried foods, including chips, French fries, and donuts

- Beverages with added sugars, like soda, energy drinks, and sweet tea

The Glucose Goddess Method is a great way to keep your blood sugar steady while enjoying the foods you love. You can promote stable blood glucose levels by emphasizing healthy carbohydrates, lean proteins, and healthy fats while avoiding processed foods with added sugars or preservatives. Plus, by eliminating deep-fried and sugary snacks from your diet, you'll be on the path to better overall health in no time! Happy eating!

MEAL PLANNING AND PORTION CONTROL

The Glucose Goddess Method is a meal planning and portion control approach that balances blood sugar levels and promotes overall health. While I don't have specific information about the Glucose Goddess Method, I can provide some general tips on meal planning and portion control that may be helpful.

1. Include a balance of macronutrients: When planning your meals, include a balance of carbohydrates, proteins, and fats. This can help stabilize blood sugar levels and provide sustained energy throughout the day.
2. Choose complex carbohydrates: Opt for whole grains, legumes, fruits, and vegetables. These foods are digested more slowly, gradually releasing glucose into the bloodstream and preventing spikes in blood sugar levels.
3. Prioritize lean proteins: Include lean protein sources in your meals, such as skinless poultry, fish, tofu, beans, or lentils. Protein helps promote satiety and can prevent overeating.
4. Incorporate healthy fats: Include sources of healthy fats in your meals, such as avocados, nuts, seeds, and olive oil. These fats provide essential nutrients and can help you feel satisfied after meals.
5. Control portion sizes: Portion control is essential for maintaining a balanced diet. Use measuring cups, a

food scale, or visual cues (e.g., using your hand as a guide) to ensure you consume appropriate portions. It's also important to listen to your body's hunger and fullness cues to avoid overeating.

6. Eat smaller, frequent meals: Some people find it helpful to eat smaller, more frequent meals throughout the day to maintain steady blood sugar levels. This can help prevent energy crashes and excessive hunger.

7. Plan and prepare meals in advance: Set aside sometime each week to plan and prepare your meals. This can help you make healthier choices and avoid relying on processed or fast foods when you're short on time.

8. Stay hydrated: Drinking enough water is important for overall health and can help control appetite. Aim to drink water throughout the day and limit sugary beverages.

Remember, it's always a good idea to consult a registered dietitian or nutritionist who can provide personalized guidance based on your specific dietary needs and health goals. They can help tailor a meal plan and portion control strategy that aligns with the Glucose Goddess Method or any other dietary approach you follow.

CHAPTER 5:

EXERCISE AND PHYSICAL ACTIVITY

THE IMPACT OF EXERCISE ON BLOOD SUGAR

Exercise significantly impacts blood sugar levels, particularly for individuals with diabetes. Here are some key ways in which exercise affects blood sugar:

1. Increased glucose uptake: During exercise, your muscles require energy to perform physical activity. They take up glucose from the bloodstream, even without insulin. This can lead to a decrease in blood sugar levels.
2. Improved insulin sensitivity: Regular exercise can enhance insulin sensitivity, so your body becomes more efficient at using insulin to transport glucose from the bloodstream into cells. This can help

lower blood sugar levels and improve overall glycemic control.

3. Reduced insulin resistance: Insulin resistance is a condition where the body's cells become less responsive to the effects of insulin. Regular physical activity can reduce insulin resistance, making it easier for insulin to regulate blood sugar levels effectively.

4. Temporary increase in blood sugar levels: Intense or prolonged exercise can cause a temporary increase in blood sugar levels. This happens due to the release of stress hormones, such as adrenaline, which stimulate the liver to release stored glucose into the bloodstream. This effect is more common in individuals without diabetes or those not properly managing their blood sugar levels.

5. Post-exercise blood sugar drop: After exercising, blood sugar levels can sometimes drop below normal levels, a condition called hypoglycemia. This can occur within a few hours following physical activity and may

be more common in individuals who take insulin or certain diabetes medications. Monitoring your blood sugar levels after exercise and adjusting your medication or food intake if necessary is important.

6. Individual variability: The impact of exercise on blood sugar can vary depending on factors such as the type, intensity, and duration of the activity, as well as individual factors like fitness level, medication regimen, and overall health. Monitoring your blood sugar levels before, during, and after exercise is important to understand how your body responds.

For individuals with diabetes, it's crucial to work closely with healthcare professionals, such as doctors and certified diabetes educators, to develop an exercise plan that considers individual needs and goals. They can provide personalized guidance on adjusting medication, monitoring blood sugar, and managing potential exercise-related fluctuations in blood sugar levels.

EXERCISE SIGNIFICANTLY IMPACTS BLOOD SUGAR

Levels, particularly for individuals with diabetes. Here are some key ways in which exercise affects blood sugar:

1. Increased glucose uptake: During exercise, your muscles require energy to perform physical activity. They take up glucose from the bloodstream, even without insulin. This can lead to a decrease in blood sugar levels.
2. Improved insulin sensitivity: Regular exercise can enhance insulin sensitivity, so your body becomes more efficient at using insulin to transport glucose from the bloodstream into cells. This can help lower blood sugar levels and improve overall glycemic control.
3. Reduced insulin resistance: Insulin resistance is a condition where the body's cells become less responsive to the effects of insulin. Regular physical activity can reduce insulin

resistance, making it easier for insulin to regulate blood sugar levels effectively.

4. Temporary increase in blood sugar levels: Intense or prolonged exercise can cause a temporary increase in blood sugar levels. This happens due to the release of stress hormones, such as adrenaline, which stimulate the liver to release stored glucose into the bloodstream. This effect is more common in individuals without diabetes or those not properly managing their blood sugar levels.

5. Post-exercise blood sugar drop: After exercising, blood sugar levels can sometimes drop below normal levels, a condition called hypoglycemia. This can occur within a few hours following physical activity and may be more common in individuals who take insulin or certain diabetes medications. Monitoring your blood sugar levels after exercise and adjusting your medication or food intake if necessary is important.

6. Individual variability: The impact of exercise on blood sugar can vary depending on factors such as the type, intensity, and duration of the activity, as well as individual factors like fitness level, medication regimen, and overall health. Monitoring your blood sugar levels before, during, and after exercise is important to understand how your body responds.

For individuals with diabetes, it's crucial to work closely with healthcare professionals, such as doctors and certified diabetes educators, to develop an exercise plan that considers individual needs and goals. They can provide personalized guidance on adjusting medication, monitoring blood sugar, and managing potential exercise-related fluctuations in blood sugar levels.

CREATING AN EXERCISE ROUTINE

Creating an exercise routine involves considering your fitness goals, preferences, and available time. Here are some steps to help you develop an effective exercise routine:

1. Define your goals: Determine what you want to achieve through exercise. Your goals could be improving cardiovascular fitness, increasing strength, losing weight, reducing stress, or combining. Setting specific, measurable, attainable, relevant, and time-bound (SMART), goals will help guide your routine.
2. Assess your current fitness level: Evaluate your fitness level to determine your starting point. Consider factors such as cardiovascular endurance, strength, flexibility, and balance. This assessment will help you choose appropriate exercises and track your progress.
3. Choose activities you enjoy: Select exercises and activities that you genuinely enjoy. This increases the likelihood of sticking to your routine long-term. Options may include

walking, jogging, cycling, swimming, dancing, weightlifting, yoga, or group fitness classes. Varying your routine can keep it interesting and prevent boredom.

4. Determine frequency and duration: Decide how many days per week you can commit to exercise. The American Heart Association recommends at least 150 minutes of moderate-intensity aerobic activity or 75 minutes of vigorous-intensity aerobic activity per week and muscle-strengthening activities at least two days per week. Break down your exercise sessions into manageable durations based on your schedule and fitness level.

5. Plan your workouts: Create a weekly schedule that includes specific exercises, their duration, and their intensity level. Include cardiovascular exercises (such as brisk walking or jogging) and strength-training exercises (using bodyweight, free weights, or resistance machines). It's also beneficial to incorporate

flexibility exercises like stretching or yoga. Gradually increase the intensity or duration of your workouts over time to challenge yourself and continue making progress.

6. Warm-up and cool down: Before each exercise session, warm up your muscles with light cardio activity (e.g., brisk walking) and perform dynamic stretches. Cooling down after exercise allows your heart rate and breathing to return to normal gradually and can include static stretches.

7. Listen to your body: How your body feels during and after exercise. If you experience pain, dizziness, or other unusual symptoms, modify or stop the activity. Working within your limits and gradually progressing to avoid injury is important.

8. Stay consistent: Consistency is key to achieving results. Make exercise a regular routine and prioritize it like any other important commitment. Find ways to stay motivated, such as working out with a friend, joining a

class, tracking your progress, or rewarding yourself for reaching milestones.

Remember to consult your healthcare provider before starting any new exercise program, especially if you have any underlying health conditions or concerns. They can provide personalized recommendations and ensure your exercise routine meets your needs and abilities.

CHAPTER 6:

STRESS MANAGEMENT AND BLOOD SUGAR

UNDERSTANDING THE STRESS-BLOOD SUGAR CONNECTION

Stress can significantly impact blood sugar levels, especially for individuals with diabetes. Here's an explanation of the stress-blood sugar connection:

1. Stress response and hormones: When you experience stress, your body releases stress hormones, such as cortisol and adrenaline. These hormones prepare your body for a "fight-or-flight" response, which includes raising blood sugar levels to provide extra energy to deal with the perceived threat.
2. Increased glucose production: Stress hormones stimulate the liver to release stored glucose into the bloodstream. This glucose is meant

to provide energy for immediate use in response to the stressful situation.

3. Insulin resistance: Stress hormones can also lead to temporary insulin resistance. Insulin regulates blood sugar levels by helping glucose enter cells to be used as energy. When insulin resistance occurs, cells become less responsive to insulin, and glucose remains in the bloodstream, leading to higher blood sugar levels.

4. Emotional eating and food choices: Many people turn to food for comfort or stress relief, which can impact blood sugar levels. During stressful periods, some individuals may overeat or choose high-sugar, high-calorie comfort foods, which can cause blood sugar spikes.

5. Disrupted routines: Stress can disrupt regular routines, including meal planning, exercise, and medication adherence. Inconsistent eating patterns missed medications, or decreased physical activity can all

contribute to fluctuations in blood sugar levels.

For individuals with diabetes, managing stress and blood sugar levels is crucial. Here are some

Strategies to help mitigate the impact of stress on blood sugar:

- Practice stress management techniques: Engage in stress-reducing activities such as deep breathing exercises, meditation, yoga, or hobbies you enjoy. Regular exercise can also help reduce stress levels.
- Plan healthy meals and snacks: Maintain a balanced diet focusing on whole foods, including lean proteins, complex carbohydrates, and healthy fats. This can help stabilize blood sugar levels even during stressful periods.
- Establish consistent routines: Stick to regular meal times, medication

schedules, and exercise routines as much as possible. Consistency can help promote stable blood sugar levels.

- Seek social support: Connect with supportive friends, family, or support groups to discuss your stressors and share coping strategies. Having a support system can help reduce the impact of stress on your overall well-being.
- Monitor blood sugar levels: Regularly check your blood sugar levels during stressful periods to identify patterns or changes. This information can help you make necessary adjustments to your diabetes management plan.

If you find that stress consistently impacts your blood sugar levels or if you're having difficulty managing stress, it's important to consult with your healthcare provider or a mental health professional. They can provide guidance, support, and additional strategies to manage stress effectively and maintain optimal blood sugar control.

STRESS REDUCTION TECHNIQUES

Managing stress is essential for overall well-being, and numerous techniques can help reduce stress levels. Here are some effective stress reduction techniques you can try:

1. Deep Breathing: Practice deep breathing exercises to promote relaxation. Breathe deeply through your nose, hold for a few seconds, and exhale slowly through your mouth. Focus on the sensation of your breath and let go of tension with each exhale.
2. Meditation and Mindfulness: Engage in mindfulness meditation to bring your attention to the present moment and cultivate a sense of calm. Find a quiet space, sit comfortably, and focus on your breath or a specific object. Allow thoughts to come and go without judgment.
3. Physical Exercise: Regular physical activity can help reduce stress and improve mood. Choose activities you

enjoy, such as walking, jogging, swimming, dancing, or yoga. Exercise releases endorphins, which are natural mood-boosting hormones.

4. Progressive Muscle Relaxation (PMR): PMR involves tensing and relaxing different muscle groups to release physical tension and promote relaxation. Start with your toes and work through your legs, abdomen, arms, and face.

5. Engage in Hobbies: Pursuing activities you enjoy can provide a sense of joy and help distract from stressors. Whether painting, playing a musical instrument, gardening, reading, or cooking, allocate time for hobbies that bring you pleasure and relaxation.

6. Social Support: Reach out to friends, family, or support groups for emotional support. Talking about your stressors, sharing experiences, and receiving empathy can help alleviate stress. Maintain social connections through in-person or virtual interactions.

7. Time Management: Effective time management can reduce stress caused by feeling overwhelmed or rushed. Prioritize tasks, break them into smaller, manageable steps, and set realistic deadlines. Use tools like calendars or to-do lists to stay organized.

8. Healthy Lifestyle Habits: Adopting a healthy lifestyle can improve your coping skills. Sleep well, eat a balanced diet, limit caffeine and alcohol intake, and avoid smoking. Taking care of your physical well-being can positively impact your mental and emotional well-being.

9. Relaxation Techniques: Explore other relaxation techniques such as aromatherapy, listening to calming music, taking a warm bath, or practicing yoga or Tai chi. Find activities that help you unwind and promote a sense of tranquility.

10. Seek Professional Help: If stress becomes overwhelming or persistent, consider seeking help from a mental health professional. They can provide

guidance, support, and additional strategies tailored to your needs.

Remember, what works for one person may not work for another. Experiment with different techniques and find a combination that suits you best. Consistency and regular practice are key to experiencing the benefits of stress reduction techniques.

INCORPORATING MINDFULNESS AND RELAXATION PRACTICES

Incorporating mindfulness and relaxation practices into your daily routine can reduce stress and promote overall well-being. Here are some ways to incorporate these practices into your life:

1. Start with a few minutes each day: Begin by setting aside just a few minutes for mindfulness and relaxation. This can be in the morning, during a break at work, or before bed. As you become more

comfortable, gradually increase the duration of your practice.

2. Mindful breathing: Take a few moments to focus on your breath. Close your eyes and bring your attention to the sensation of your breath as you inhale and exhale. Let go of distracting thoughts and observe your breath as it naturally flows in and out.

3. Body scan meditation: Lie down or sit comfortably and bring your attention to different body parts, starting from your toes and moving up to the top of your head. Notice any sensations or areas of tension, and consciously release any tension or tightness as you focus on each body part.

4. Mindful eating: Slow down and fully engage your senses while eating. Notice the colors, textures, smells, and flavors of your food. Take your time to chew slowly and savor each bite. Pay attention to your body's hunger and fullness cues.

5. Walking meditation: Take a mindful walk outdoors, paying attention to

the sensations in your body as you move. Feel the ground beneath your feet, notice the rhythm of your steps, and observe the sounds and sights around you. If your mind wanders, gently bring your focus back to the present moment.

6. Guided meditation apps or recordings: Use guided meditation apps or online recordings to provide structured mindfulness and relaxation practices. These resources offer a variety of guided sessions, making it easier to get started and maintain regular practice.

7. Yoga or tai chi: Engage in yoga or tai chi, which combines mindful movement with breath awareness. These practices help cultivate a sense of calm, improve flexibility, and promote relaxation. Attend classes or follow online tutorials to learn and incorporate the techniques into your routine.

8. Mindfulness reminders: Use daily reminders or cues to bring mindfulness into everyday activities.

For example, you can set a reminder on your phone to pause and take a few deep breaths every hour or place sticky notes with mindfulness quotes in visible areas.

9. Create a calming environment: Set up a designated space in your home where you can practice mindfulness and relaxation. Decorate it with soothing colors, candles, cushions, or anything that helps create a serene atmosphere.

10. Integrate mindfulness into daily tasks: Bring mindfulness to your daily activities, such as washing dishes, showering, or brushing your teeth. Focus on these activities' sensations, movements, and sounds rather than being on autopilot.

CHAPTER 7:

LIFESTYLE MODIFICATIONS FOR BALANCED BLOOD SUGAR

SLEEP AND BLOOD SUGAR REGULATION

Too little sleep can also affect blood sugar regulation, and people with diabetes are particularly vulnerable. Studies have shown that people who get an average of four or fewer hours of sleep per night are more likely to experience problems with their glucose levels. The Glucose Goddess Method emphasizes the importance of getting enough sleep and eating healthy meals and snacks throughout the day to keep blood sugar levels in a normal range. Adequate rest is necessary for optimal health, so ensure you get at least seven to eight hours of quality sleep each night. In addition, following a balanced diet low in added sugars and high in fiber-rich foods can help regulate blood sugar levels naturally. Finally, regular exercise is essential for maintaining healthy blood sugar levels, so prioritize an active lifestyle. Following the Glucose Goddess Method can help you stay on track and better manage your diabetes.

This is especially important during times of stress, such as when going through an illness or dealing with changes in the environment that may affect glucose levels. Ensuring adequate sleep, following a balanced diet, and exercising regularly will help maintain optimal glucose control. With discipline and guidance from the Glucose Goddess Method, you'll be well on your way toward managing your diabetes effectively.

HYDRATION AND BLOOD SUGAR HEALTH

Hydration plays a crucial role in maintaining blood sugar health. Here's how hydration can affect blood sugar levels:

1. Blood sugar dilution: Staying properly hydrated helps to maintain adequate blood volume and prevents blood from becoming too concentrated. When dehydrated, your blood becomes more concentrated, leading to higher blood sugar levels. Drinking enough water helps dilute the blood, ensuring better blood sugar control.
2. Kidney function: The kidneys are vital in filtering waste products, including glucose, from the blood. When you're well-hydrated, your kidneys can function optimally and efficiently remove excess glucose from the bloodstream. Inadequate hydration can impair kidney function, potentially affecting blood sugar regulation.
3. Digestion and nutrient absorption: Hydration is essential for proper digestion and nutrient absorption. When you consume food, the body breaks down carbohydrates into glucose, which enters the bloodstream. Sufficient hydration

supports the digestive process, ensuring efficient absorption of nutrients from the gastrointestinal tract, including glucose.

4. Exercise performance: Staying hydrated is particularly important during exercise. Physical activity can affect blood sugar levels, and dehydration can exacerbate these effects. Proper hydration before, during, and after exercise helps maintain optimal blood sugar control during physical activity.

To promote hydration and support blood sugar health, consider the following tips:

1. Drink adequate water: Aim to drink enough water throughout the day to maintain hydration. While individual needs vary, a general guideline is to consume about 8 cups (64 ounces or 2 liters) of water daily. Adjust your intake based on activity level, climate, and personal needs.

2. Limit sugary drinks: Be mindful of your beverage choices and avoid or

minimize sugary drinks such as soda, fruit juices, and sweetened beverages. These can cause blood sugar spikes and do not contribute to proper hydration. Opt for water, herbal tea, or unsweetened beverages instead.

3. Monitor urine color: Use the color of your urine as a hydration indicator. Ideally, it should be pale yellow or straw-colored. Dark-colored urine is a sign of dehydration, and you should increase your fluid intake.

4. Consider electrolytes: Electrolytes are minerals (e.g., sodium, potassium) that help maintain fluid balance in the body. You may need to replenish electrolytes if you engage in prolonged or intense exercise or have specific medical conditions. Electrolyte-rich beverages, foods, or electrolyte supplements can help in these cases.

5. Personalize your hydration plan: Age, activity level, climate, and individual health conditions can influence your hydration needs. Work with your

healthcare provider or a registered dietitian to determine the appropriate hydration plan for your unique circumstances

STRATEGIES FOR LONG-TERM SUCCESS

The Glucose Goddess Method provides a comprehensive approach to achieving and sustaining a healthy lifestyle. The strategies outlined here can help make it easier to stick with the program over the long term:

• Create an action plan. Make a detailed plan outlining how you will gradually incorporate changes into your life. Start small by making simple changes like adding more fruits and vegetables to your diet or reducing added sugars and processed foods, then slowly add in more exercise and other lifestyle modifications as you become comfortable with them.

• Set realistic goals. Don't try to do too much at once or set overly ambitious goals; aim for progress rather than perfection.

• Track your progress. Keeping track of your progress can help you stay motivated and on track with the program. Use a food diary to log meals and snacks, record the minutes you spend exercising, or use online tracking tools available through the Glucose Goddess program.

• Celebrate small successes. Instead of focusing on negative thoughts, celebrate each success - no matter how small - as it will help build momentum for future improvements.

• Get support. An experienced coach or mentor can guide and encourage to keep going when times are tough. The Glucose Goddess Method also offers forums where users can connect with people who share similar experiences and goals for motivation and camaraderie.

By following these strategies, anyone can successfully implement the Glucose Goddess Method and make positive changes to their lifestyle that will last. You can lead a healthier life today with proper guidance, commitment, and dedication.

CHAPTER 8: TROUBLESHOOTING AND DEALING WITH CHALLENGES

HANDLING BLOOD SUGAR FLUCTUATIONS

- Fluctuating blood sugar levels occur when there is an overdose of diabetes medications. For example, if a patient is on insulin, administrating insulin at the same site can cause hypertrophy of Lipohyde hypertrophy and dystrophy of the tissues, leading to high glycaemic variability. Similarly, using improper insulin administration techniques can cause high blood glucose fluctuation.
- We usually monitor glycosylated hemoglobin (HVAC), FBS & PLBS; if it is under control, we think he is out of danger and will not have any

complications. But studies say that even after maintaining Hbac FBS and PUBS if the patient has high glycaemic variability and time in range is out of control, he will land into microvascular and macrovascular complications.

It Can Be Prevented Through:

1. Dietary and lifestyle modification will help in controlling fluctuating blood sugars
2. Adequate sleep
3. Reducing weight or maintaining proper weight
4. Decreasing stress levels
5. Reduced intake of tea and coffee
6. Reduced alcohol intake
7. Proper medications
8. Regularly check-ups with primary care physician
9. Encourage taking complex carbohydrates and limiting the intake of simple carbohydrates.
10. Carbohydrate intake estimation to be done (consult with a dietician)

11. Insulin-dependent patients need to be educated about Insulin site rotation and administration technique, as improper insulin administration can also cause high glycaemic variability.
12. Chronic liver and kidney disease problems must be treated accordingly to reduce fluctuation.
13. Daily physical activity 30-45 min/day. Six days a week helps in stimulating insulin and controlling blood sugar levels.
14. Blood and urinary tract infections can also cause blood glucose fluctuations. But, again, treating infections empirically and based on culture and sensitivity will help control fluctuations.

The continuous glucose monitoring system is the most Innovative method available to diagnose significantly fluctuating blood sugar or high glycaemic variability. It has a small sensor that is attached to the body. This sensor helps monitor glucose levels from 5 to 14 days, which helps calculate glycaemic variability and time in range.

COPING WITH CRAVINGS AND TEMPTATIONS

Coping with cravings and temptations is a common challenge when maintaining a healthy lifestyle. Here are some strategies to help you navigate and manage cravings effectively:

1. Identify triggers: Become aware of the situations, emotions, or thoughts that trigger cravings. By recognizing your triggers, you can develop strategies to address them proactively. For example, if stress triggers cravings, you can implement stress-management techniques to reduce the urge to indulge in unhealthy foods.
2. Practice mindful eating: Before giving in to a craving, pause and practice mindful eating. Ask yourself if you're truly hungry or if the craving is driven by something else, such as boredom

or emotions. Slow down and savor each bite, paying attention to the taste, texture, and satisfaction you derive from the food. Mindful eating helps you become more attuned to your body's signals and make conscious choices.

3. Find healthier alternatives: Look for healthier alternatives that can satisfy your cravings. For example, if you're craving something sweet, choose fresh fruit or a small portion of dark chocolate instead of sugary snacks. Experiment with healthier recipes or find healthier substitutes for your favorite indulgent foods. This way, you can satisfy your cravings while making healthier choices.

4. Plan your meals and snacks: Establishing a meal plan and sticking to regular eating patterns can help prevent excessive hunger and minimize impulsive food choices. Plan balanced meals and include satisfying snacks to keep you satisfied throughout the day. Having nutritious options readily available

can reduce the likelihood of giving in to unhealthy cravings.

5. Practice portion control: If you're tempted by less healthy foods, practice portion control. Allow yourself to enjoy a small serving of the food you're craving rather than completely depriving yourself. You can satisfy your craving without derailing your overall healthy eating habits by savoring a small portion.

6. Distract yourself: When a craving strikes, find a distraction to redirect your attention. Engage in activities that keep your mind and body occupied, such as walking, reading a book, listening to music, or engaging in a hobby. The craving will often pass as you shift your focus to something else.

7. Stay hydrated: Sometimes, thirst can be mistaken for hunger or cravings. Ensure you stay hydrated throughout the day by drinking enough water. Before reaching for a snack, have a glass of water and see if the craving subsides.

8. Seek support: Reach out to a friend, family member, or support group for encouragement and accountability. Sharing your struggles and successes with someone who understands can provide valuable support when facing cravings and temptations.

9. Practice self-care: Taking care of your overall well-being can help reduce cravings. Prioritize sleep, manage stress, engage in regular physical activity, and practice relaxation techniques. When you prioritize self-care, you're less likely to turn to food to cope with emotional or physical discomfort.

CONCLUSION

The Glucose Goddess Method offers a comprehensive approach to managing blood sugar levels and promoting overall well-being. This method provides a holistic framework for achieving optimal health through its emphasis on meal planning, portion control, exercise, stress reduction, and mindfulness.

By adopting the principles of The Glucose Goddess Method, individuals can take control of their health and cultivate a positive relationship with their bodies. The method encourages mindful choices, empowering individuals to make informed nutrition, exercise, and overall lifestyle decisions.

Focusing on balance, self-compassion, and realistic goal setting, The Glucose Goddess Method recognizes that health is a lifelong journey. It embraces the understanding that setbacks and cravings are a normal part of the process and provides strategies for coping effectively.

Ultimately, The Glucose Goddess Method is about managing blood sugar levels and creating a fulfilling and sustainable lifestyle. It is about nourishing the body and the mind, fostering overall well-being, and finding joy in pursuing a healthy life.

So, whether you're seeking to improve your blood sugar control, enhance your physical fitness, or adopt healthier habits, The Glucose Goddess Method offers a practical and empowering approach that can guide you toward a healthier, happier, and more vibrant life.

Made in United States
Troutdale, OR
04/01/2024

18872568R00049